the teacher appears

WITH ORIGINAL CONTRIBUTIONS FROM

Mayim Bialik · Beryl Bender Birch · Rachel Brathen
Elena Brower · J. Brown · Mallika Chopra
Seane Corn · Tiffany Cruikshank · Govind Das
Krishna Das · Lori Deschene · Alan Finger
Ana T. Forrest · Sharon Gannon · Joseph Goldstein
Schuyler Grant   Anna Guest-Jelley · Dan Harris
Bryan Kest · Jack Kornfield · Tias Little
Sarah Platt-Finger · Shiva Rea · Dave Romanelli
Gretchen Rubin · Mark Stephens · David Swenson
Ganga White

the teacher
appears

108 PROMPTS TO POWER
YOUR YOGA PRACTICE

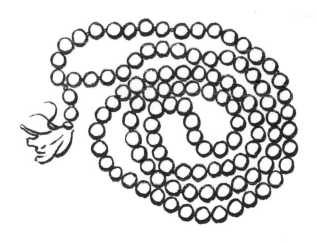

by Brian Leaf

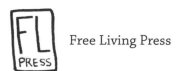

Free Living Press

Free Living Press
269 Main Street
Northampton, MA 01060
www.teacherappears.net

Ordering Information:
Quantity sales. Special discounts are available on quantity purchases. For details, contact the publisher at the address above or call 413-584-0075 or visit www.teacherappears.net.

Leaf, Brian.
The teacher appears: 108 prompts to power your yoga practice /
Brian Leaf.
ISBN 978-0692770580
1. Yoga. 2. Journal writing. 3. Health. I. Title. II. Leaf, Brian.

First Edition
ISBN 978-0692770580
Printed in the United States
10 9 8 7 6 5 4 3 2 1

Illustrations: Génévieve May, Jaclyn Whalen
Cover design: Valerie Reiss, Rebecca Neimark, Jaclyn Whalen
Interior design: Jaclyn Whalen, Rebecca Neimark

Place this book next to your yoga mat while you practice. Tuck it under your cushion while you meditate Ask your yoga teacher to bless it. Infuse and invest its pages with good vibes, until it becomes a talisman of transformation—until, when you see it or hold it, you drop instantly into your heart.

ACKNOWLEDGMENTS

Deep gratitude to my teachers, colleagues, and friends Mayim
Bialik, Beryl Bender Birch, Rachel Brathen, Elena Brower,
J. Brown, Mallika Chopra, Seane Corn, Tiffany Cruikshank,
Govind Das, Krishna Das, Lori Deschene, Alan Finger, Ana T.
Forrest, Sharon Gannon, Joseph Goldstein, Schuyler Grant,
Anna Guest-Jelley, Dan Harris, Bryan Kest, Jack Kornfield,
Tias Little, Sarah Platt-Finger, Shiva Rea, Dave Romanelli,
Gretchen Rubin, Mark Stephens, David Swenson, and
Ganga White for their generous contributions. You'll find
their original guest prompts interspersed every few pages
throughout this book.

Thanks to Dobra Tea, Esselon Café, and Amherst Coffee, where
the rest of this book was written. Thanks to Jaclyn Whalen and
Rebecca Neimark for their inspired design, to Jean Zimmer for
a super mindful edit, to Génévieve May for inking my words
into pictures, and to Georgie von Furth, my research assistant
and marketing guru. Deep gratitude also to Matthew Andrews
and Yoga Center Amherst for inspiration; to Matt Oestreicher
and the Society for Free Living for keeping me on track; to
Julie, Larry, Susan and Manny Leaf for everything; and to
Gwen, Benji, and Noah for time and the most important
ingredient of all, love. And speaking of love, this book is
dedicated, as always, to my teacher, Swami Kripalu.

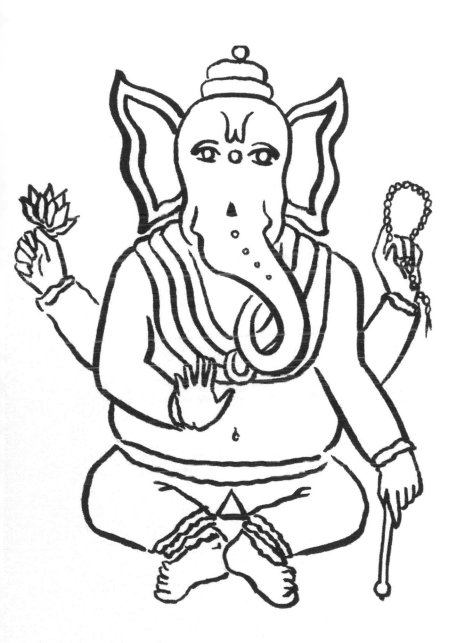

Color in Ganesha, remover of obstacles,
patron of letters and learning, god of beginnings.

Mahatma Gandhi said,

"I shall cease to be useful as soon as I cease to be myself."

Carry this journal today
and list the moments
when you are most yourself.

_____

_____

_____

_____

_____

_____

_____

Why do you do yoga? ✳

✳ Be honest. There's no wrong answer.

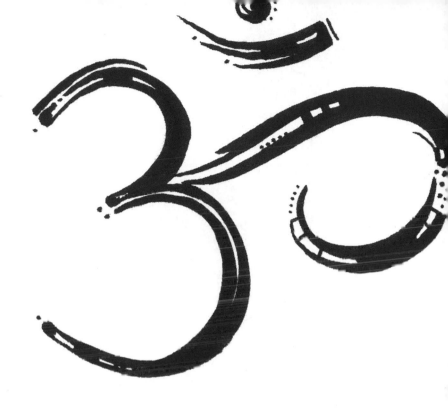

Set a timer on your phone and chant "om"

slowly and repeatedly for 5 minutes.

ANNA GUEST-JELLEY
FOUNDER OF CURVY YOGA

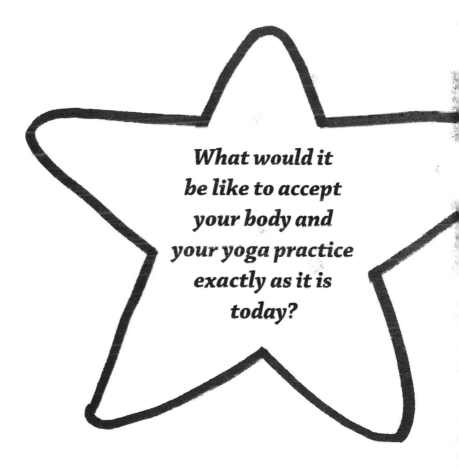

*What would it
be like to accept
your body and
your yoga practice
exactly as it is
today?*

Live into that answer today on your mat.

Break the bonds of mindless
habit. Close this book and go
do the most unlikely thing.

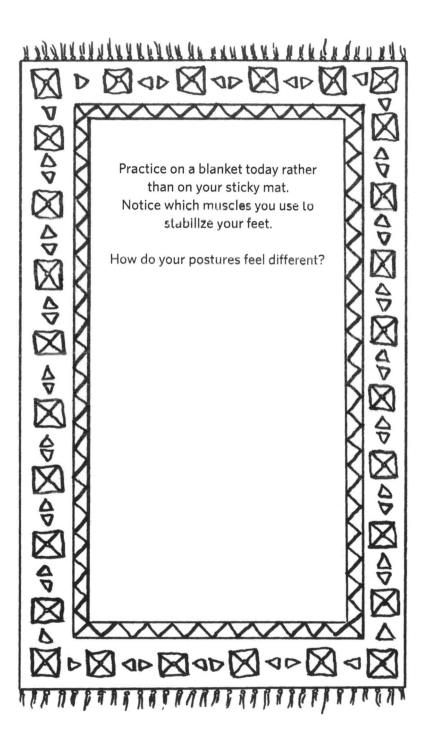

Practice on a blanket today rather
than on your sticky mat.
Notice which muscles you use to
stabilize your feet.

How do your postures feel different?

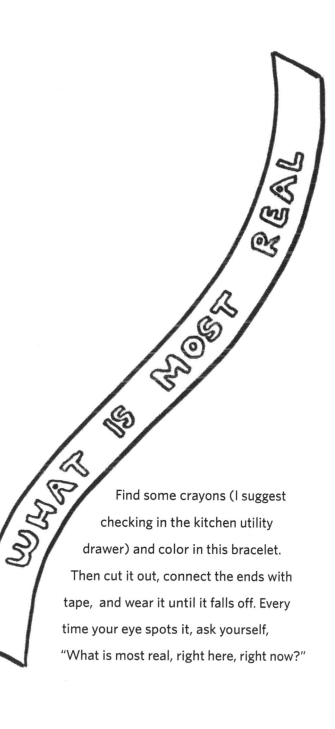

WHAT IS MOST REAL

Find some crayons (I suggest checking in the kitchen utility drawer) and color in this bracelet. Then cut it out, connect the ends with tape, and wear it until it falls off. Every time your eye spots it, ask yourself, "What is most real, right here, right now?"

What part of your body **IRKS** you the most?

_____

_____

_____

_____

Send ridiculous amounts of love and kisses and tenderness
there right now and during your next yoga practice.

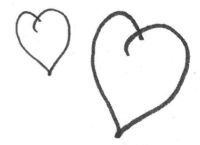

JOSEPH GOLDSTEIN,
MEDITATION TEACHER AND AUTHOR OF
MINDFULNESS: A PRACTICAL GUIDE TO AWAKENING

The erroneous belief that genuine happiness comes only from pleasant feelings can become a strong motivation to stay closed to anything unpleasant. But by staying closed to all unpleasantness, we also stay closed to our own wellspring of compassion.

Can you mindfully open today to one unpleasantness that you typically avoid?

How does your yoga practice connect you to others?

_____

_____

_____

_____

_____

How does it separate you?

_____

_____

_____

_____

_____

Complete this sentence:

I have known for a while now that it is time for me to _____

_____

_____

_____

_____

Sit up tall and then mentally state,

May I be happy. May I be well.
May I know that I belong.
May I be peaceful and at ease.

Then bring to mind a friend or loved one,
close your eyes, and mentally state,

May you be happy. May you be well.
May you know that you belong.
May you be peaceful and at ease.

Repeat this for another loved one or friend,
closing your eyes and mentally stating,

May you be happy. May you be well.
May you know that you belong.
May you be peaceful and at ease.

Now bring to mind someone with whom
you have difficulty, and mentally state,

May you be happy. May you be well.
May you know that you belong.
May you be peaceful and at ease.

Then relax, breathe deeply, and open your eyes.

How do you feel? _____

_____

_____

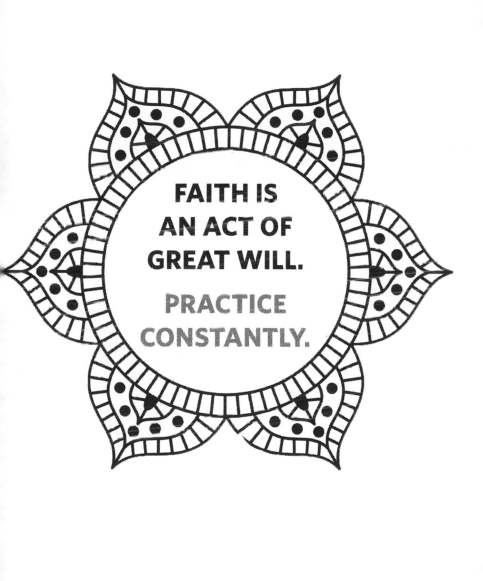

FAITH IS
AN ACT OF
GREAT WILL.

PRACTICE
CONSTANTLY.

GOVIND DAS
COFOUNDER OF
BHAKTI YOGA SHALA

Bring your hands to the prayer position in front of your chest. Go deep into your heart, your deepest and innermost spiritual heart, and with total sincerity and clarity finish the following statement:

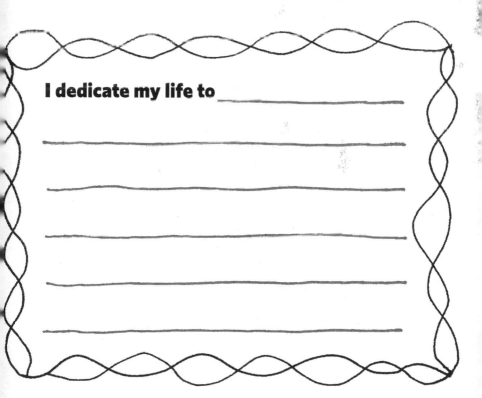

I dedicate my life to _____

Meditation 101. Sit up tall and turn your attention to the natural inhalation and exhalation of breath. Notice the rise and fall of the belly or the sensation of breath passing through the nostrils. Anytime your mind wanders, return your awareness to the breath. That's it. Try it now for 5 minutes.

Draw pictures of your mind
before and after your next meditation.

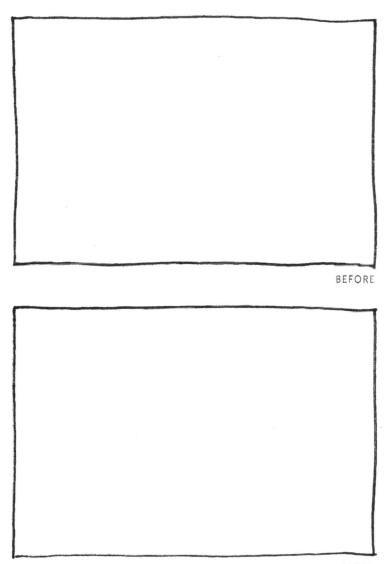

BEFORE

AFTER

Set a timer and spend 3 minutes without talking, looking into the eyes of a friend or partner. *How do you feel afterward?*

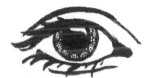 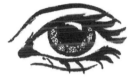

Just once, fart loudly during a yoga class.

☑

1.12.17

Check box when completed.

Bring this book into nature and sit
next to a tree or a calm body of water.

Notice how you feel.

Is your mind jumpy or relaxed?
Is your breathing calm or quick?

Sit until you settle and catch the calm vibe of nature.

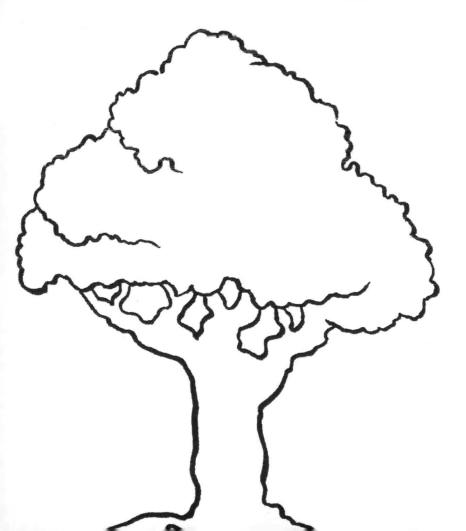

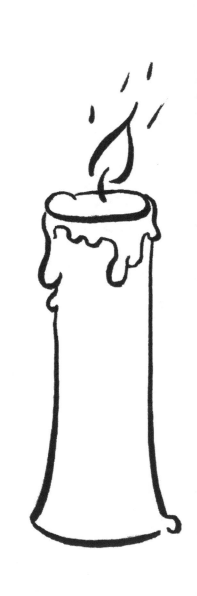

1. Set your alarm for 5:30 a.m.

2. In the morning, light candles and practice gentle, sacred yoga.

3. Feel the deep peace of the early morning.

Afterward, journal below.

_____

_____

_____

_____

_____

_____

_____

_____

_____

BERYL BENDER BIRCH
DIRECTOR/FOUNDER OF
THE HARD & THE SOFT YOGA INSTITUTE
AND THE GIVE BACK YOGA FOUNDATION

Sit for 10 minutes. Back straight. Close your eyes.
Be still. Notice your breath. Drop in on this moment.
No agenda, no fanfare, not trying to get anywhere.
Just be present. Fully here. Fully awake. What do you
notice? Sensation? Sound? Thought? If you get carried
downstream on some long narrative, just notice.

Come back. No thinking about thinking. Just this.

Stand up, legs together, and place this book between your thighs. Use your core muscles to move the book backward and forward. **Practice until you can do it smoothly.**

Like this

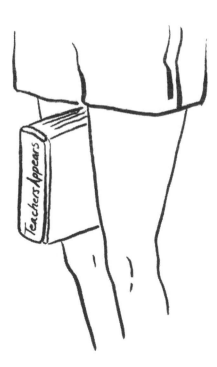

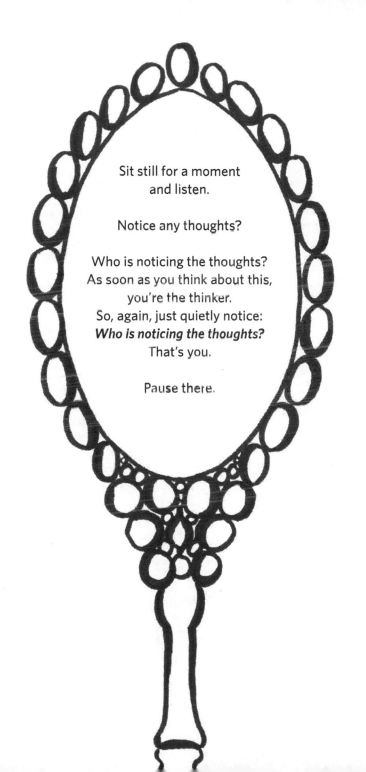

Sit still for a moment
and listen.

Notice any thoughts?

Who is noticing the thoughts?
As soon as you think about this,
you're the thinker.
So, again, just quietly notice:
Who is noticing the thoughts?
That's you.

Pause there.

GRETCHEN RUBIN,
AUTHOR OF *THE HAPPINESS PROJECT*
AND *BETTER THAN BEFORE*

Look up at the sky. Notice the colors, the clouds, the quality of the light, perhaps the leaves and buildings against the sky. **Really look.**

In the space below, describe what you see— in words or in images.

Find a photo of a saint, a very small statue of the Buddha, or
any such sacred object that appeals to you. **Sketch it below.**

Tuck the sacred object into your pocket and hold it every time
you make a decision today.

DAVID SWENSON
ASHTANGA YOGA TEACHER

There are fears that keep us alive and fears that keep us from living.

Wisdom is to understand the difference.

List five fears that serve you.

1. _____

2. _____

3. _____

4. _____

5. _____

List five fears you can release.

1. _____

2. _____

3. _____

4. _____

5. _____

DAN HARRIS
AWARD-WINNING ABC NEWS ANCHOR
AND AUTHOR OF *10% HAPPIER*

Promise yourself that for the next 2 weeks you'll meditate for 10 minutes every day, wherever you can—in your bedroom, your office, or your car (as long as you're not driving). In fact, set a daily reminder on your phone. And set another reminder to come back to this page in 2 weeks.

After 2 weeks, are you doing better at responding wisely to situations in your life rather than reacting blindly?

☐   ☐
YES   NO

Good. Keep it going!

For the rest of the day, every time you hear a smartphone **beep** or **buzz,** stop whatever you are doing and take a deep, mindful breath.

Balance
this
book
on
your
head
during
tadasana
(mountain
posture)
today.

Ask yourself
In this moment, what is lacking?
What is keeping me from feeling completely at ease?
Explore. Look within. The answer might surprise you.

No lies today.
See how it feels.

Rip this page out and
tuck it into your pocket
so you'll remember.

As you practice yoga today, bring your awareness to where in your body you most feel each posture. After each posture, in one of the diagrams below, **color in the places of greatest sensation.**

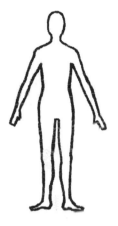

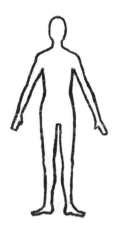

POSTURE _____   POSTURE _____

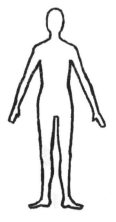

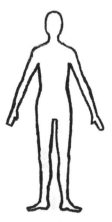

POSTURE _____   POSTURE _____

JACK KORNFIELD
MEDITATION TEACHER,
AUTHOR OF *A PATH WITH HEART*

When you find yourself in difficulty or in conflict,
whether in a conversation, an e-mail, or a text message,
pause, take a breath, and ask your heart
What is my highest intention?

Notice how your words and tone change.

Make a list of people who deeply love you.

Hold your list. Soak it in.
Carefully tear out this page and slip it into your datebook,
or take a photo of it and set it as wallpaper
on your home screen.

GANGA WHITE
AUTHOR OF *YOGA BEYOND BELIEF,*
FOUNDER OF THE
WHITE LOTUS FOUNDATION

Yoga doesn't take time; it gives time.

Try this 7-Day Yoga Challenge:
Practice for at least 15 minutes every day this week and see if
it makes you feel more or less harried and rushed.

Check off each day as you meet the challenge.

☐ **Monday**

☐ **Tuesday**

☐ **Wednesday**

☐ **Thursday**

☐ **Friday**

☐ **Saturday**

☐ **Sunday**

Focusing your gaze focuses the mind. Experiment with *drishti* (focused gaze) during yoga postures today. During each posture, choose a point of focus (such as your thumb, your toes, or a distant point on the wall or floor).

How does this alter your practice?

Focus here

Meditate in the following times, places, or ways.
(Check off when complete.)

☐ *Right before bed*

☐ *First thing in the morning*

☐ *At work*

☐ *At a relative's home*

☐ *With a partner or friend*

☐ *In a city*

☐ *Near a waterfall*

☐ *At a state or national park*

☐ *In a holy place*

☐ *On top of a mountain*

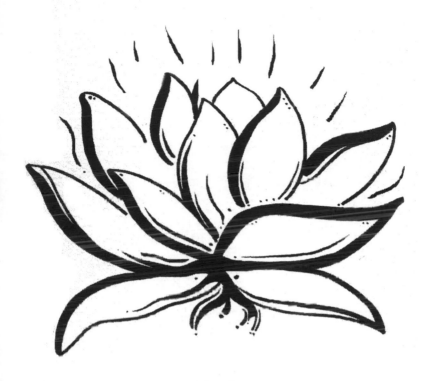

Visualize

a white lotus flower

behind your belly button.

Picture it radiant,

shining

with a bright light.

Meditate on this flower for 5 minutes.

MAYIM BIALIK
EMMY AWARD NOMINEE FOR
THE BIG BANG THEORY,
AUTHOR OF *BEYOND THE SLING*
AND *MAYIM'S VEGAN TABLE*

For today, when you practice yoga, let go of the need
to get it "right" as well as the need to keep up with or
outdo the person next to you.

Instead, allow your yoga today to be exactly what it is.

Record your results below.

_____

_____

_____

_____

_____

_____

_____

Take a break right now, set a timer on your phone for
5 minutes, and practice alternate nostril breathing.

Alternate Nostril Breathing 101. Sit up tall and, using your
right hand, close off your right nostril with your thumb as you
inhale slowly through the left nostril. Then close off your left
nostril with your ring finger and exhale slowly through the
right. Then inhale slowly through the right, switch fingers,
and exhale slowly through the left. Repeat this for 5 minutes.

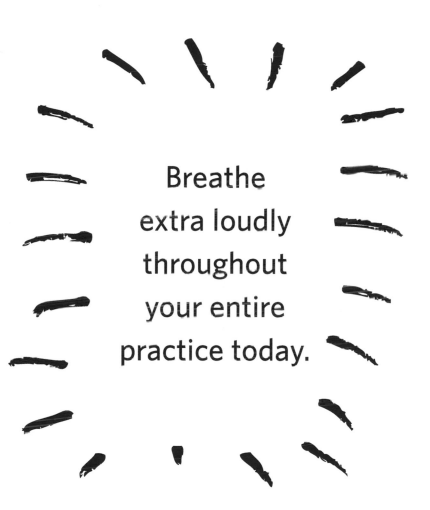

Breathe
extra loudly
throughout
your entire
practice today.

Add chanting to your postures. While you hold each yoga posture, slowly and deeply chant the sound of the area where you most feel the stretch. (See the chart below. Each *aaa* is vocalized like the *o* in *Tom*.)

FEET, LEGS, PERINEUM	"LAAAMM"
PELVIS, HIPS	"VAAAMM"
BELLY, LOW BACK	"RAAAMM"
CHEST, UPPER BACK	"YAAAMM"
NECK, SHOULDERS	"HAAAMM"

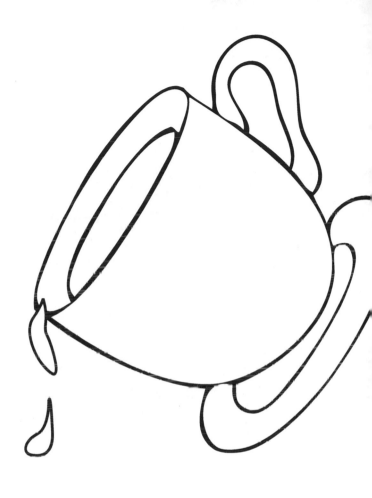

**Ask someone
from yoga class out
to tea or for a walk.**

ELENA BROWER
COAUTHOR OF *ART OF ATTENTION:*
A YOGA PRACTICE WORKBOOK
FOR MOVEMENT AS MEDITATION

What is your practice helping you understand about your family?

The next time you practice postures or meditation at
home, place this book, along with a pen, beside you.
When you're done, do some freewriting.
Don't even think about what you're writing.
Just let it spill out.

Describe your very first yoga class. *What do you remember?*

_____

_____

_____

_____

_____

When did you fall In love with yoga?

_____

_____

_____

_____

_____

List fifty things for which you are grateful.
See if you can do it in one writing session.
Practice until you can.

Just for today, no complaining about anything.
Speak only gratitude.
Keep this book with you so you'll remember.

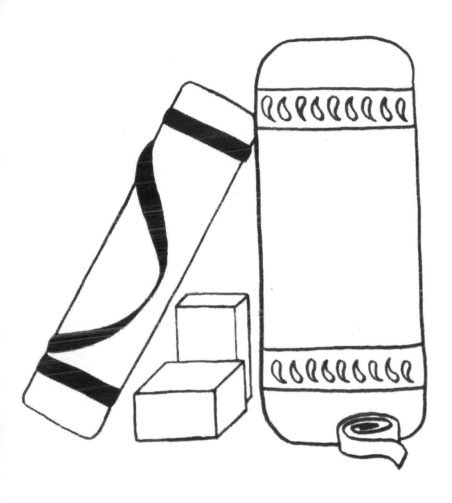

Use props in your yoga practice today.
Include this book as a block so you won't forget.

MALLIKA CHOPRA
AUTHOR OF *LIVING WITH INTENT,*
FOUNDER OF INTENT.COM

> *"You are what your deepest desire is. As your desire is, so is your intention. As your intention is, so is your will. As your will is, so is your deed. As your deed is, so is your destiny."*

—Upanishads

What is your deepest desire?

Every time you speak today, place your hand on your heart.

(Probably best done on a day off from work.)

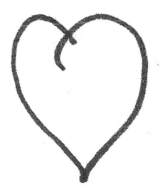

After your practice today, carefully tear out this page
and write a note to someone you love.
Then decorate the page and mail it.

Dear _____,

I love you. _____

_____

_____

_____

_____

_____

_____

_____

_____

Love, _____

ANA T. FORREST
MEDICINE WOMAN,
CREATRIX OF FORREST YOGA,
AUTHOR OF *FIERCE MEDICINE*

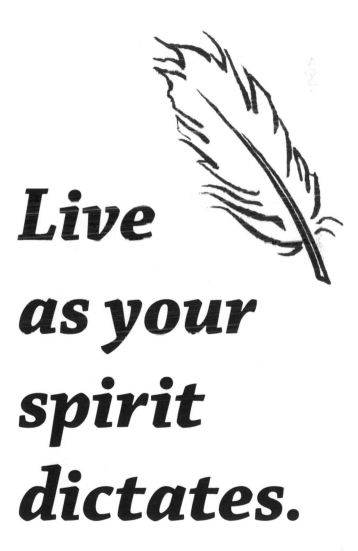

*Live
as your
spirit
dictates.*

Reclaim consciousness from the mind.
Right now, for 10 seconds, drop your awareness into your
body and experience the world directly through your senses.

  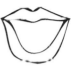

List three people you resent.

1 _____

2 _____

3 _____

Forgive them now. This is true yoga.

MARK STEPHENS
AUTHOR OF *YOGA SEQUENCING:*
DESIGNING TRANSFORMATIVE YOGA CLASSES

If you want to go deep,
go slow.

Stretch the breath
to stretch your practice,

and open your senses
to feel it all.

List four health rules you follow quite strictly.

1 _____

2 _____

3 _____

4 _____

Choose one to break tomorrow.

Set up a yoga altar. You can use a crate, a footstool, a shoe box, or a gold and a marble pedestal. It can be in a corner of your bedroom or office or under the shoe rack in your walk-in closet. On your altar, place special stones, a candle, a statue or image of a spiritual teacher, a representation of God, or a photo of a deceased loved one. After you finish reading this paragraph, close your eyes and see what your altar looks like. Don't dream it up; just look in your mind's eye and see what's already there.

Draw a picture of your altar here.

What about yourself have you repressed to "fit in"?
What have you given up?

Claim it back now.

Krishna Ram Shiva
haShem The Light
Elohim El-Shaddai
Vishnu Jesus Allah
Yahweh Jehovah
Adonai Christ Ram
Ar-Rahman Khuda
Huwa Krishna Shiva
Bhagavan Brahma
Satnam Great Spirit

KRISHNA DAS
KIRTAN WALLAH,
DEVOTEE OF NEEM KAROLI BABA

Chanting the Names of God will dissolve our false sense of separateness and allow us to lose our small self in the Ocean of Love, which is our True Nature.

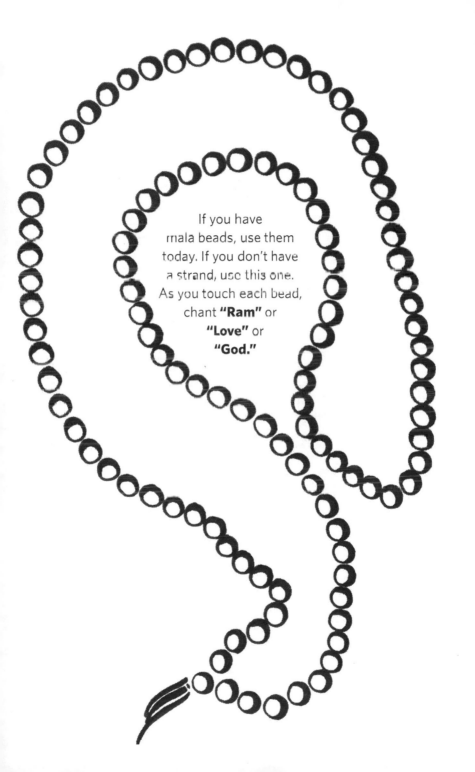

If you have mala beads, use them today. If you don't have a strand, use this one. As you touch each bead, chant **"Ram"** or **"Love"** or **"God."**

Choose someone in class

and secretly send them

good vibes.

What are your five favorite postures?

1 _____

2 _____

3 _____

4 _____

5 _____

Do a whole yoga practice today
with only these five postures,
and then tomorrow
do a full practice without them.

Choose a half day and do *only* what brings you joy.
This may be harder than it sounds.

Record the date here:

_____

When was the last time you stole something?
Was it an object or an idea? Apologize below.
Then gently rip out this page, ceremonially burn it, let it go,
and forgive yourself. Your yoga will be deeper for it.

SEANE CORN
YOGA TEACHER, ACTIVIST,
AND COFOUNDER OF
OFF THE MAT, INTO THE WORLD

Stand in front of your mat and dedicate every movement of today's practice to someone you love, someone who needs healing, or someone you need to forgive. Notice if it changes the way you move, the way you breathe, or the way you feel.

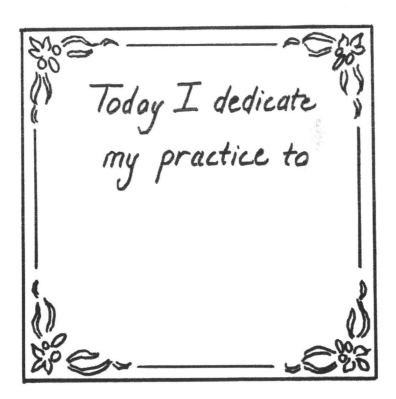

Today I dedicate my practice to

TAKE A BREAK. PLAY. GET
THE ENERGY FLOWING. PUT
ON SOME MUSIC. DANCE. SING.
FROLIC. MAYBE FIND A FRIEND
AND ENJOY A CAREFUL GAME
OF CATCH WITH THIS BOOK.
KEEP COUNT AND SEE IF YOU
CAN GET TO TWENTY-FIVE
WITHOUT DROPPING IT.

This

month,

when

you are

flipping

through

Yoga

Journal,

actually read the articles.

Allow yourself to long for God.

Do it now.

List as many of your yoga teachers as you can remember.

Describe each teacher's style.

J. BROWN
FOUNDER OF ABHYASA YOGA CENTER

How do you feel right now?

Internally repeat the words *I rock*.
Notice any change?

Repeat the phrase at least fifty more times today (particularly
at moments of difficulty) and watch what happens.
Begin now.

Spend a half-day in silence.

Cut out the following signs. Post one on your front door and wear the other as a necklace. You provide the string.

String goes here

Today I am taking a half-day of silence

from _____ to _____ .

Please come back at _____ .

Thank you!

String goes here

Today I am taking a half-day of silence

from _____ to _____ .

Please come back at _____ .

Thank you!

For today, ask yourself, with every important action, *Why am I doing this?* No judgment, only awareness. Keep a log below.

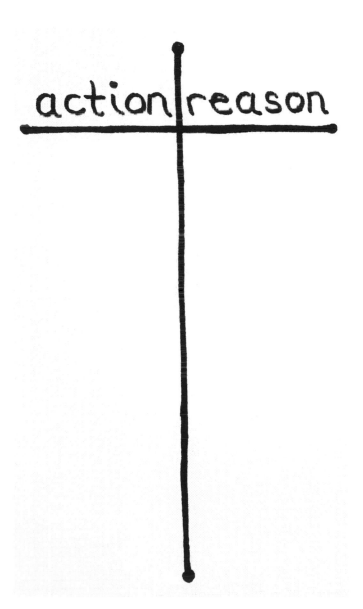

action|reason

"Better is one's own dharma [essential nature or duty], though imperfectly carried out, than the dharma of another carried out perfectly."

—Bhagavad Gita

What is your dharma?

Write a letter to your future self.
Any advice? Reminders? Questions?

Dear _____ ,

[your name here]

_____

_____

_____

_____

_____

_____

_____

_____

_____

Over

→

_____

_____

_____

_____

_____

_____

_____

_____

_____

_____

Love, _____

[your name here]

Good. Now rip out this page and mail it to yourself. But use
the wrong house number and the wrong zip code so it takes
longer to get to you.

Spend a week as a yoga tourist. Try a class
in a different style or even at a different studio.
Can you follow the instructions and lingo?
What does it feels like to be an outsider?

Record your impressions below.

SHIVA REA
AUTHOR OF *TENDING THE HEART FIRE:*
LIVING IN FLOW WITH THE PULSE OF LIFE

Pause, and connect to
your heart center.
How can you circulate
more love within and to
all living beings?

TIAS LITTLE
FOUNDER OF PRAJNA YOGA,
AUTHOR OF *YOGA OF THE SUBTLE BODY*

Carry this book and record five times this week when your blood pressure rises—on your mat, stalled in traffic, attending a meeting, or visiting a family member. **What happens in your gut, your jaw? How does it affect your breathing?**

1. _____

2. _____

3. _____

4. _____

5. _____

Just by noticing, you can begin to release the pressure.

Do everything different in class today.
If you're always the last to release a posture, be the first.
If you usually give up early, hold it longer.
If you sit in the back, move to the front.
Chant a little louder or quieter.
Ask a question today, or don't ask any.
Wear sweatpants instead of yoga pants, or vice versa.

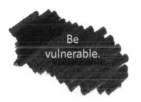

Close this book now
and share deeply with someone you love.

After you read this page, close your book and practice one simple act of selfless giving.

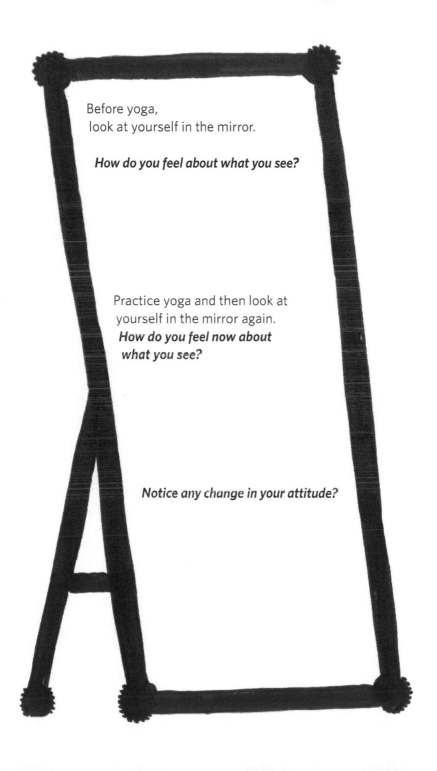

Before yoga,
look at yourself in the mirror.

How do you feel about what you see?

Practice yoga and then look at
yourself in the mirror again.
*How do you feel now about
what you see?*

Notice any change in your attitude?

Are you the same person in yoga class and at work?

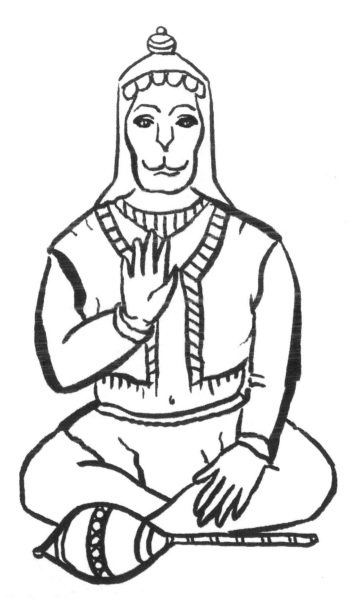

Color in Lord Hanuman, the monkey god,
a symbol of strength, energy, and unyielding devotion.

Teach yourself
a new posture
from a book.
I recommend
B.K.S Iyengar's
Light on Yoga.

Do your postures in a TIGHT SPACE today. Maybe in the dining room or a walk-in closet.

What five tips would you give to a beginner?

1. _____

_____

2. _____

_____

3. _____

_____

4. _____

_____

5. _____

_____

Are these the same five tips you wish
someone had given you before your first class?

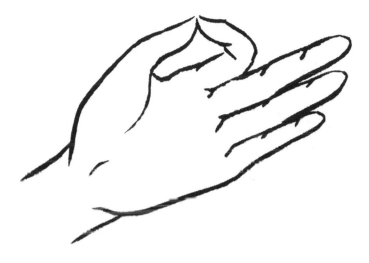

Try adding mudra to your practice. When possible,
while holding each posture, touch your index finger
to your thumb to make Gyan Mudra.

How does it feel? **Record results below.**

BRYAN KEST
FATHER OF POWER YOGA,
CREATOR OF WESTERN
DONATION-BASED YOGA

The harder you are on anything, the faster you wear it out.

Be gentle.

Do you unconsciously use any habit—such as overeating, oversocializing, getting drunk, binging on Netflix, or picking a fight with a friend or partner—to dissipate your energy after a great yoga class?

See if you can catch yourself next time and, instead, hold the high, if even for just an extra hour.

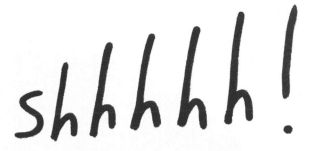

shhhhh!

Try to go a full day without telling anyone anything about yoga. **How does it feel?**

SCHUYLER GRANT

DIRECTOR OF KULA YOGA PROJECT,
CO-FOUNDER OF THE WANDERLUST FESTIVAL

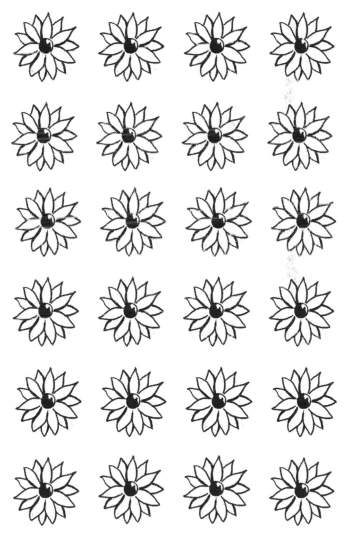

Beginner's mind never grows old.

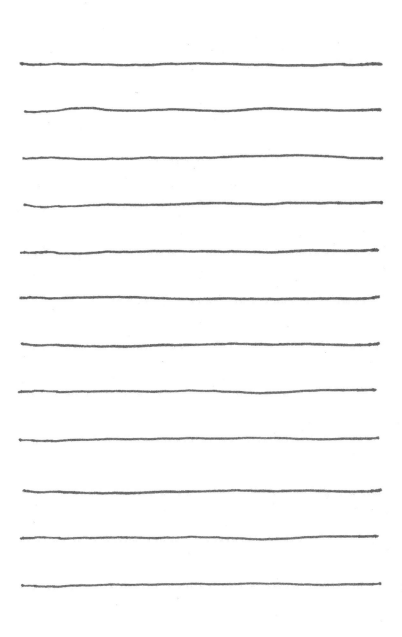

Fill all the lines below as you describe something amazing.
You can use a tree, a stone, a loving touch, a knitted sweater,
or a flourless chocolate torte. Describe every nuance
and detail. **Use all your senses.**

Fill both pages

TIFFANY CRUIKSHANK
FOUNDER OF YOGA MEDICINE

When you move through your practice today, approach each pose as if it were your medicine. Notice whether you are taking the proper dosage. *Are you holding a pose for too long or not long enough?* **How does your practice feel different with this mental shift?**

Write yourself a yoga prescription below.

R͟X *Yoga Prescription*

Name: _____

INSTRUCTIONS:

SIGNATURE: DATE:

Forgive the tightness in your hamstring and it will ease.

Try this now.

"In the silence of the heart God speaks."

–Mother Teresa

Relax your body. Sit quietly. Breathe.
In the silence of the moments
between breaths, **listen.**

What do you hear?

SHARON GANNON
CO-FOUNDER OF JIVAMUKTI YOGA

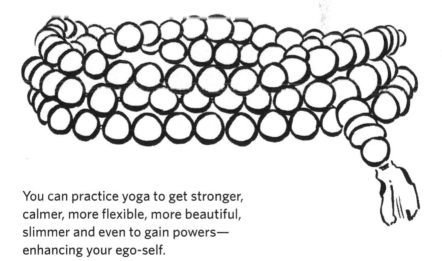

You can practice yoga to get stronger,
calmer, more flexible, more beautiful,
slimmer and even to gain powers—
enhancing your ego-self.

The wise are humble and practice yoga
to realize Yoga—their connection to God.

Bring this journal to a crowded place. Look around for a few moments and see everyone as the tip of an iceberg. See each person's iceberg extending deep below. See all the huge icebergs connected at their bases.

Draw what you see.

ALAN FINGER AND
SARAH PLATT-FINGER
COFOUNDERS OF ISHTA YOGA

Feel the moment between two thoughts,
which is the pause between two breaths.

This is pure consciousness.

 Set a reminder on your phone to notice this
at the top of every hour.

> **"Your task is not to seek for love, but merely to seek and find all the barriers within yourself that you have built against it."**
>
> —Rumi

How do you get in the way of love?

Clean your bedroom today. But here's the catch.
As you tidy up, hold each item in your hands. If the item
sparks joy, keep it. Otherwise, chuck it. It's gone.
We shall never speak of it again.

Identify five pieces of clutter in your family room or office
and to whom you will gift them.

Note: The recycling bin or dumpster is a
perfectly viable recipient.

Place a check mark in front of each one when completed.

☐ 1. _____

_____

☐ 2. _____

_____

☐ 3. _____

_____

☐ 4. _____

_____

☐ 5. _____

_____

There are three ways to be in the world:

1. To believe that we are each alone and separate from one another.

2. To realize that we are all connected.

3. To realize that we are all one.

—Ram Dass

Which way do you live?

LORI DESCHENE
FOUNDER OF TINYBUDDHA.COM,
AUTHOR OF *TINY BUDDHA'S*
365 TINY LOVE CHALLENGES

Take your flexibility off the mat today. If things don't go as planned, ask yourself:

How can I embrace what is and even make the most of it?

What would it look like to let go of control and let life happen?

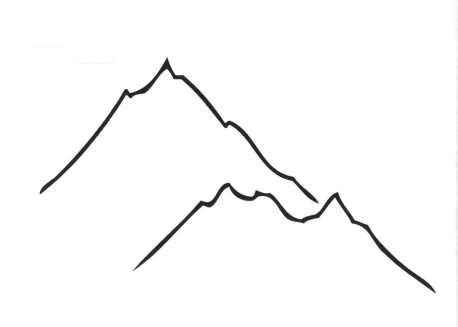

Climb a mountain until you have an expansive view.
Breathe deeply and ask for guidance.

What do you receive?

DAVE ROMANELLI
AUTHOR OF
HAPPY IS THE NEW HEALTHY

Skip yoga today and enjoy a super long *savasana*
(yogic relaxation).

Afterward, eat exotic chocolate.

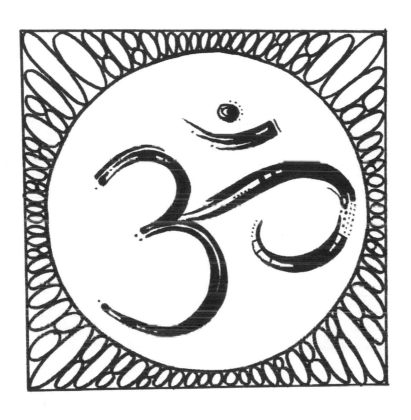

Color in this om, a representation of God,
the original sound and most sacred mantra.

BRIAN LEAF is the author of thirteen books, including *Misadventures of a Garden State Yogi*. Brian graduated from Georgetown University in 1993 with a BA in business, English, and theology, and in 1999 he completed a master's degree at Lesley College, specializing in yoga and ayurveda. He lives in Northampton, Massachusetts, with his wife and two sons. Brian is a devotee of Swami Kripalvananda.

ALSO BY BRIAN LEAF

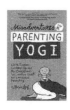

Misadventures of a Parenting Yogi: Cloth Diapers, Cosleeping, and My (Sometimes Successful) Quest for Conscious Parenting

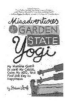

Misadventures of a Garden State Yogi: My Humble Quest to Heal My Colitis, Calm My ADD, and Find the Key to Happiness